FATTY LIVER DIET COOKBOOK

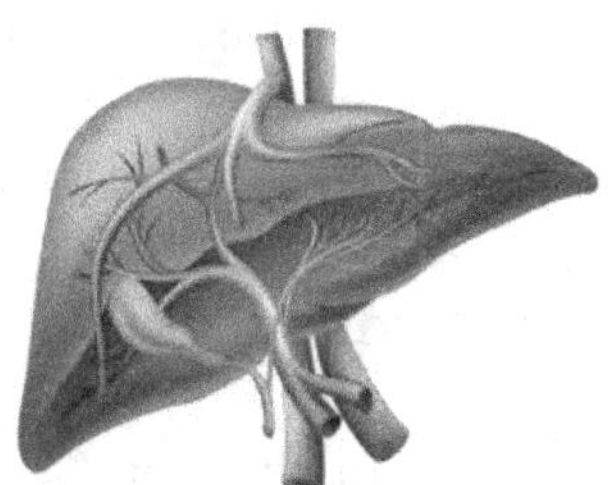

A Comprehensive Guide with Quick, Tasty and Healthy Recipes to Detoxify and Revitalize Your Liver, Increase Energy and Weight loss

Andrew Fred

Copyright © 2024 by Andrew Fred

TABLE OF CONTENTS

My Liver Disease Story Experience

Once upon a time, in a little village set amid rolling hills, lived James, a joyful guy whose laughter boomed through the local tavern. His evenings were punctuated by clinking glasses and the camaraderie that only a close-knit community could deliver. Yet, little did he realize, his passion for the amber liquid was slowly exacting a toll on his liver.

One regular examination altered the path of James' life. The early diagnosis sent shockwaves through him—a warning message from his liver, highlighting the repercussions of continued alcohol consumption.

The doctor's sharp remarks were a wake-up call, a sobering revelation that led James to reassess his lifestyle choices.

Determined to restore his health, James dove into the realm of liver-friendly foods and meal planning. Armed with a renewed resolve, he adopted the Fatty Liver Diet Cookbook as his guide.

The process began with comprehending the nuances of fatty liver disease and the impact his diet had on its progression. It was a voyage of self-discovery, realizing the need for change and finding peace in the healing power of nutritious, nutrient-rich meals.

The fundamental guide to a healthy liver lifestyle became James' blueprint, and he navigated the chapters with attention.

He devised culinary remedies that not only tantalized his taste buds but also nursed his diseased liver. Meal planning became an art—a conscious effort to design each dish with elements that supported healing and energy.

In the course of weeks, James observed a tremendous metamorphosis. The modest transition from damaging food habits to a nutritious culinary excursion was like a salve for his liver.

The support of the Fatty Liver Diet Cookbook, together with his persistence, resulted in a reversal of the preliminary stage of liver disease.

As James relished his newfound health, he became a beacon of hope for those suffering from similar illnesses. To people standing at the crossroads of change, he sent a message of perseverance and optimism. Every recipe, every meal, and every constructive choice was a step toward recovery.

For the diagnostic patients still in the basic stages of liver illness, James' experience became a testament to the transformational potential of a conscious diet.

The Fatty Liver Diet Cookbook, once his ally in recovery, now stood as a beacon of hope, blazing the route toward a better destiny. It whispered the promise that, with devotion and the correct decisions, they too could rewrite the story of their health, flipping the page to a brighter, more vibrant chapter.

INTRODUCTION

As we live in a society where the decisions we make about our nutrition have a significant impact on our overall health, the incidence of fatty liver disease has become an urgent matter of concern. The condition known as fatty liver disease, which is defined by the accumulation of extra fat in the cells of the liver, does pose a substantial threat to our general health. When excessive fat deposits penetrate the liver, it becomes damaged.

The liver is a powerful organ that is responsible for digesting nutrients and cleansing the body throughout this process. Because fatty liver disease is a quiet condition and has the potential to have long-term effects on one's health, it is necessary to have a thorough understanding of its severity.

From the mildest types of fatty liver to its most severe manifestations, this problem requires our attention and compels us to take preventative measures for the management of that condition.

A strong ally in the fight against fatty liver disease is the role of nutrition, which stands out among the array of instruments that are available for making this fight possible. The decisions that are made regarding one's diet have a significant impact, not only on the acceleration of the disease but also on the prevention of it.

Through the adoption of a diet that is beneficial to the liver, one may reduce the dangers connected with fatty liver disease and pave the way for a life that is healthier and fuller of vitality.

It is with this awareness and devotion to health that the "Fatty Liver Diet Cookbook" emerges as a wonderful resource. This cookbook is not simply a collection of recipes; rather, it is an all-encompassing handbook that is intended to inspire individuals on their journey toward liver health.

The recipes on these pages are meticulously designed to delight the taste buds and nourish the liver, combining ingredients renowned for their therapeutic benefits for liver health.

As we begin this gastronomic excursion, let us understand the significance of our dietary choices in defining the destiny of our livers. The "Fatty Liver Diet Cookbook" is more than a tool for cooking meals; it is a guide to a lifestyle that celebrates health, welcomes balance, and supports the complex dance between nutrition and well-being.

Together, let us take care of our liver health and begin on a tasty journey toward a future distinguished by energy and enduring well-being.

CHAPTER 1

Understanding Fatty Liver Disease

In the complicated fabric of human health, the liver appears as a quiet sentinel, persistently executing crucial processes to maintain our bodies in harmony. However, when faced with the development of fatty liver disease, this tenacious organ is thrown into the forefront, demanding our attention and care.

Understanding Fatty Liver Disease

Fatty liver disease, a disorder defined by the excessive accumulation of fat in liver cells, can present in numerous forms, ranging from benign fatty liver to the more dangerous non-alcoholic steatohepatitis (NASH). To embark on the road toward liver wellness, it is vital to know the subtleties of this condition.

From its mild beginnings to potential problems, having awareness of fatty liver disease serves as the foundation for educated decision-making in the quest for a healthy liver lifestyle.

The Fatty Liver Diet: Basics

At the root of controlling and preventing fatty liver disease lies the power of diet. The Fatty Liver Diet, anchored on principles of balance and moderation, is the bedrock of our fight against this frequent ailment. Embracing nutrient-dense meals while reducing the intake of processed and sugary treats becomes vital. Understanding the foundations of this diet empowers individuals with the tools needed to make conscious dietary choices, supporting liver health and general well-being.

The Fatty Liver Diet Cookbook

A culinary companion on the path to liver health, the "Fatty Liver Diet Cookbook" serves as a tribute to the transformational potential of well-crafted meals.

Within its pages, a multitude of dishes awaits, each devised with the twin objective of exciting taste buds and nourishing the liver. From morning treats to delicious meals and seductive sweets, the cookbook transcends every day, enabling readers to appreciate the delicacies of a liver-friendly lifestyle.

Lifestyle Changes for a Healthy Liver

Beyond the sphere of the kitchen, genuine liver health is created through comprehensive lifestyle adjustments. Physical exercise, stress management, and frequent health check-ups are key components of a routine geared toward developing a robust liver.

This chapter dives into the symbiotic link between lifestyle choices and liver well-being, giving practical insights for developing a holistic approach to a healthy liver lifestyle.

As we embark on this journey through the essential guide, let us fortify our understanding of fatty liver disease, embrace the fundamentals of the Fatty Liver Diet, explore the delectable offerings within the cookbook, and set the stage for transformative lifestyle changes that will pave the way toward a life marked by a resilient and thriving liver.

CHAPTER 2

Culinary Solutions for Fatty Liver Wellness

In the area of fatty liver wellness, the road toward vibrant health unfolds not only in the choices we make within the kitchen but also in the tremendous influence our culinary selections have on our entire well-being.

Fatty Liver Disease: Unveiling the Mystery

Before we continue on our gastronomic voyage, it is necessary to reveal the enigma of fatty liver disease. This chapter aims to demystify this ailment, diving into its different manifestations, causes, and the complicated dance between lifestyle and liver health. By unlocking the riddle, we empower ourselves with knowledge, developing a proactive approach in the face of this ubiquitous and often insidious condition.

Forms of Fatty Liver Disease

1. Non-Alcoholic Fatty Liver (NAFL)

This frequent form of fatty liver disease is defined by the buildup of fat in the liver cells in people who do not use excessive alcohol. It frequently presents as a benign disorder but can escalate to more severe phases.

2. Non-Alcoholic Steatohepatitis (NASH)

NASH is a more advanced stage of fatty liver disease, defined by inflammation and liver cell destruction. Unlike NAFL, NASH can lead to problems such as fibrosis, cirrhosis, and, in certain circumstances, liver failure.

3. Alcoholic Fatty Liver Disease (AFLD)

Excessive alcohol use can result in the buildup of fat in the liver cells. AFLD varies from a basic fatty liver to more serious diseases, including alcoholic hepatitis and cirrhosis.

Causes of Fatty Liver Disease

1. Dietary Factors

Consuming a diet heavy in saturated fats, sweets, and processed foods contributes greatly to the development of fatty liver disease. Poor dietary choices can lead to an imbalance in lipid metabolism and fat buildup in the liver.

2. Obesity

Excess body weight, particularly abdominal obesity, is a key risk factor for fatty liver disease. Obesity impairs normal metabolic processes, resulting in fat buildup in the liver.

3. Insulin Resistance and Type 2 Diabetes

Insulin resistance, commonly linked with type 2 diabetes, leads to the development of fatty liver disease. Elevated insulin levels induce fat accumulation in the liver.

4. Genetic Factors

Some individuals may be genetically prone to fatty liver disease. Genetic differences can alter how the body processes and stores fat, impacting liver function.

Intricate Dance between Lifestyle and Liver Health

1. Physical Activity

Regular exercise has a significant role in preventing and controlling fatty liver disease. Physical activity helps increase insulin sensitivity, aids weight reduction, and lowers fat storage in the liver.

2. Nutrient-Dense Diet

Adopting a nutrient-dense diet, rich in fruits, vegetables, whole grains, and lean proteins, helps liver function. These meals contain vital vitamins, minerals, and antioxidants that help with liver function.

3. Moderation in Alcohol Consumption

For persons with alcoholic fatty liver disease, moderation or abstinence from alcohol is crucial to prevent additional liver damage.

4. Stress Management

Chronic stress can contribute to the development and progression of fatty liver disease. Implementing stress management practices, such as mindfulness and relaxation exercises, is excellent for liver function.

Understanding these varied forms and causes and the delicate interplay between lifestyle variables and liver function is crucial.

Armed with this knowledge, individuals may make educated decisions to avoid, control, and possibly reverse the symptoms of fatty liver disease, paving the way for a healthier and more resilient liver.

The Cookbook: A Gastronomic Journey to Health

Central to our culinary investigation is the "Fatty Liver Diet Cookbook." This section enables readers to embark on a culinary trip that surpasses the typical bounds of dietary restrictions. Crafted with care, the cookbook is a treasure trove of dishes meant not only to gratify the palette but also to feed the liver.

From exquisite breakfast alternatives to savory meals and luscious desserts, each recipe serves as a testament to the belief that health and cuisine can harmoniously coexist.

Mastering the Art of Meal Planning

As we navigate the landscapes of flavor and nutrition, the art of meal planning emerges as a talent of critical importance. This chapter gives practical insights into perfecting this skill, including assistance in designing weekly diet plans that promote liver health.

From recognizing nutrient-rich products to adopting successful grocery shopping tactics, readers are given the tools to weave the fabric of liver-friendly cooking practices.

Practical Insights toward Mastering Meal Planning

1. Set clear objectives

Begin by outlining the goals of your food plan. Whether it's weight control, enhanced nutrition, or specialized dietary requirements for fatty liver health, clarity on objectives leads the whole meal planning process.

2. Understand Nutrient Requirements

Tailor meal programs to satisfy the dietary needs required for liver health. This involves including the right mix of carbs, proteins, healthy fats, and necessary vitamins and minerals.

3. Embrace Variety

Ensure diversity in your meals to provide a wide range of nutrients. This not only boosts the overall nutritional profile but also makes the meal plan more pleasurable and sustainable.

4. Portion Control

Practicing portion control is vital for regulating calorie intake and reducing overeating. Be cautious of serving sizes to achieve a balance that promotes both liver function and general well-being.

5. Incorporate liver-friendly foods

Integrate foods renowned for their good influence on liver health. Include products like leafy greens, cruciferous vegetables, berries, fatty salmon, and whole grains, since these contribute to good liver function.

6. Strategic Meal Timing

Plan meals strategically throughout the day to maintain stable blood sugar levels and sustain energy levels. Aim for regular, properly spaced meals and snacks to avoid lengthy periods without nutrients.

7. Preparation and batch cooking

Streamline the meal preparation process by batch cooking and preparing items in advance. This not only saves time but also guarantees that healthy selections are easily available, eliminating the temptation for less nutritious choices.

8. Smart Grocery Shopping

Create a shopping list based on your food plan to minimize impulse purchases. Prioritize healthy, nutrient-dense meals while eliminating processed and sugary ones.

9. Flexibility and adaptability

Recognize that life comes with unexpected happenings. Design your meal plan to be flexible and adaptive, allowing for adjustments without sacrificing your overall nutritional goals.

10. Seek professional guidance

Consider talking with a nutritionist or healthcare expert, especially if you have specific dietary requirements connected to fatty liver disease. Their experience helps ensure your food plan corresponds with your health objectives.

Mastering the art of meal planning requires a combination of strategic thought, nutritional understanding, and practical application.

By incorporating these ideas into your meal planning process, you may establish a sustainable and liver-friendly strategy for fueling your body, maintaining overall health, and actively controlling fatty liver disease.

Beyond the Plate: Lifestyle and Wellness

Culinary solutions stretch beyond the plate, beyond the bounds of the kitchen, into the domain of lifestyle and well-being. This section investigates the symbiotic link between food choices, physical exercise, and stress management.

By taking a holistic approach, readers may enhance their liver wellness journey, ensuring that the benefits extend well beyond the limitations of specific meals.

As we immerse ourselves in this chapter, let us solve the complexities of fatty liver disease, relish the joys inside the cookbook, master the art of meal planning, and embrace a lifestyle that embraces the fundamental relationship between our culinary choices and general well-being.

The path to fatty liver fitness beckons, embellished with delicacies that not only delight the taste senses but also feed the body and spirit.

The goal of a healthy liver lifestyle extends far beyond the decisions made at the dining table. This section analyzes the symbiotic link between food choices, physical exercise, and stress management, exposing the interwoven dimensions of well-being.

1. Dietary Choices and Physical Activity

Dietary choices and physical exercise share a reciprocal connection, each impacting the effectiveness of the other. A nutrient-dense diet provides the energy necessary for maximum physical performance, while regular exercise boosts the body's capacity to process and absorb nutrients. Together, they constitute a powerful combination that promotes general health, including liver function.

2. Physical Activity and Liver Health

Regular physical exercise is a cornerstone of liver health. Exercise supports weight control, decreases insulin resistance, and boosts general metabolic function.

This, in turn, helps prevent and control fatty liver disease, ensuring that the liver performs at its best.

3.   Stress Management and Dietary Choices

The association between stress and eating choices is substantial. In times of stress, individuals may be prone to making less nutritious diet choices, opting for comfort foods heavy in sugars and fats. Conversely, a well-balanced diet rich in nutrients can lead to greater stress resistance.

4.   Dietary Choices and Stress Management

Certain diets, such as those high in omega-3 fatty acids and antioxidants, have been connected with stress reduction. These meals can significantly improve brain function and hormone control, helping individuals' better cope with stress. Avoiding excessive coffee and processed foods is also vital for maintaining steady energy levels and mood.

5. Integrated Lifestyle

The symbiotic link between food choices, physical exercise, and stress management stresses the significance of an integrated lifestyle strategy. Rather than seeing each part in isolation, individuals are urged to develop a holistic viewpoint, knowing that decisions made in one aspect of life can greatly influence others.

6. Positive Feedback Loop

Engaging in a healthy lifestyle produces a positive feedback loop. Improved nutritional choices can lead to higher energy levels, making physical exercise more pleasurable. Simultaneously, regular exercise can decrease stress and increase mood, producing a suitable atmosphere for maintaining good food habits.

7. Holistic Well-Being

Recognizing the interdependent nature of these lifestyle components fosters overall well-being.

This comprehensive approach not only improves liver function but also adds to total physical, mental, and emotional wellness.

Understanding and actively cultivating the synergistic link between food choices, physical exercise, and stress management is crucial. By embracing a lifestyle that harmonizes these aspects, individuals may create a robust and healthy foundation for liver health and general well-being.

CHAPTER 3

Nourishing Your Liver: A Culinary Adventure

In search of optimal liver health, go on a gastronomic adventure that exceeds the bounds of the kitchen. This chapter digs into the nuances of nourishing your liver, decoding fatty liver illness, presenting the "Fatty Liver Diet Cookbook," constructing balanced meal plans, and investigating holistic liver care that reaches well beyond the domain of culinary delights.

Decoding Fatty Liver Disease

To navigate the culinary journey effectively, it is necessary to grasp the subtleties of fatty liver disease. Understanding its different forms, causes, and the symbiotic link between lifestyle choices and liver health lays the basis for educated decision-making.

This chapter unravels the enigma of fatty liver disease, offering clarity on how dietary choices play a vital role in the prevention, treatment, and potential reversal of this widespread condition.

Understanding the delicate association between dietary choices and fatty liver disease is crucial for the prevention, treatment, and even eventual reversal of this frequent disorder. This section decodes the influence of food choices in each of these aspects:

Fatty Liver Disease Prevention

1. Nutrient-Dense Diet

Adopting a nutrient-dense diet is vital for avoiding fatty liver disease. This involves eating a mix of fruits, vegetables, nutritious grains, and lean meats. These foods include critical vitamins, minerals, and antioxidants that promote liver function and prevent the buildup of excessive fat.

2.   Balanced Macronutrients

Maintaining a balance between carbs, proteins, and lipids is crucial. Avoiding excessive consumption of refined carbs and sweets helps avoid insulin resistance, a contributing component of fatty liver disease.

3.   Hydration

Consumption helps the liver function by assisting in the detoxification process. Staying hydrated is vital for the effective metabolism of nutrients and the removal of waste products.

4.   Management

Portion Control: Controlling portion sizes helps regulate calorie intake, which is critical for people with fatty liver disease. This promotes weight control and minimizes stress on the liver.

5. Limiting Saturated and Trans Fats

Restricting the intake of saturated and Trans fats helps control fatty liver disease. These lipids can contribute to inflammation and additional liver damage.

6. Moderation in Alcohol Consumption

For persons with alcoholic fatty liver disease, moderation or abstinence from alcohol is crucial to treating the condition and preventing increasing liver damage.

7. Potential Reversal

Weight Loss: Achieving and maintaining a healthy weight is generally connected with the potential reversal of fatty liver disease. Weight loss lowers the buildup of fat in the liver and can increase insulin sensitivity.

8. Liver-Friendly Foods

Actively consuming foods known for their good influence on liver health, such as fatty fish, leafy greens, and berries, can help to the possible reversal of fatty liver disease.

9. Monitoring Sugar Intake

Limiting the consumption of added sugars and high-fructose corn syrup is vital. Excessive sugar intake has been linked to insulin resistance and the development and progression of fatty liver disease.

Understanding the multifaceted impact of dietary choices in the prevention, treatment, and potential reversal of fatty liver disease allows individuals to make educated decisions.

By adopting a liver-friendly diet that coincides with these principles, individuals may take an active part in improving the health and resilience of their livers.

Beyond the Kitchen: Holistic Liver Care

While the kitchen is an important venue in the hunt for liver health, the adventure goes beyond its limits. Holistic liver care covers lifestyle choices that improve overall well-being. From engaging in regular physical exercise that supports liver function to stress management approaches that nurture emotional equilibrium, this chapter discusses the diverse approaches needed for a robust and healthy liver.

As we immerse ourselves in this culinary adventure, let us understand the complexity of fatty liver disease, relish the joys inside the cookbook, learn the skill of making balanced meal plans, and adopt a holistic view of liver care.

Chapter 3 asks readers to not only fuel their livers but also to start on a transforming path towards robust health and well-being.

Holistic liver care extends beyond dietary choices, stressing a holistic approach to promote a robust and functioning liver. The multiple tactics included in this section include:

1.   Regular physical activity

Engaging in regular physical exercise is crucial for maintaining optimum liver function. Exercise assists in weight control, decreases insulin resistance, and boosts overall metabolic health. Incorporating a combination of aerobic activity, weight training, and flexibility exercises helps to create a holistic approach to liver care.

2.   Stress Management Techniques

Chronic stress can have harmful impacts on liver health. Implementing stress management practices, such as mindfulness, meditation, deep breathing exercises, or yoga, is vital. These techniques help manage stress hormones, ease tension, and enhance mental well-being, producing a favorable environment for liver health.

3.   Adequate Sleep

Quality sleep is vital for general health, including liver function. Aim for 7-9 hours of unbroken sleep each night.

Establishing a consistent sleep habit and generating a favorable sleep environment assist in the body's regeneration processes, promoting liver health.

4. Limiting Exposure to Toxins

Minimizing exposure to environmental contaminants is crucial for liver care. This involves limiting exposure to toxins, chemicals, and dangerous substances. Individuals may make intentional decisions such as utilizing natural cleaning products, selecting organic meals, and avoiding excessive exposure to dangerous elements in their surroundings.

5. Regular health check-ups

Regular monitoring of liver function during health check-ups is critical for the early discovery and therapy of any liver-related disorders. Routine screenings, blood tests, and meetings with healthcare specialists guarantee proactive treatment and quick intervention if needed.

6. Moderate Alcohol Consumption or Abstinence

For people with liver problems, particularly alcoholic fatty liver disease, a reduction in alcohol usage or full abstinence is necessary. Limiting alcohol intake alleviates the stress on the liver and enhances its regenerating ability.

7. Maintaining a Healthy Weight

Achieving and maintaining a healthy weight is helpful for liver function. Weight control helps minimize the risk of fatty liver disease and alleviates stress on the liver. A combination of a balanced diet and frequent physical exercise aids in maintaining a healthy weight.

8. Social Support and Mental Well-Being

Cultivating a strong social network and promoting mental well-being contribute to holistic liver care. Positive social connections and mental health practices boost overall resilience and coping skills, positively improving liver health.

By adopting these holistic techniques outside the kitchen, individuals may strengthen their livers against many stresses and create an atmosphere favorable to good liver function. This complete strategy provides a robust and healthy liver that supports overall well-being.

CHAPTER 4

Fatty Liver Diet Cookbook: A Roadmap to Wellness

Embark on a transforming journey with the "Fatty Liver Diet Cookbook," where each meal becomes a stepping stone toward a healthier, more vibrant existence. This chapter serves as your path to well-being, supporting you in creating healthy habits and continuing the trip beyond the pages of the cookbook.

Building Healthy Habits

Beyond the delightful meals, the cookbook acts as a tool for creating healthy behaviors that reach well beyond the kitchen. We delved into the art of mindful eating, portion control, and adding nutrient-dense meals into your daily routine. As you experiment with the recipes, you'll discover how to create habits that improve liver health and contribute to your overall well-being.

In the pursuit of optimal liver health and general well-being, adopting healthy behaviors is crucial. This section describes and discusses a set of practices that not only help liver health but also build a holistic sense of wellness:

1. Mindful Eating

Cultivate the practice of attentive eating by paying attention to the flavors, textures, and feelings of each mouthful. Eating deliberately and appreciating your meals helps increase digestion and establish a healthy connection with food.

2. Portion Control

Adopting portion control behaviors helps manage calorie intake and reduce overeating. Be conscious of portion sizes, listen to your body's hunger and fullness cues, and resist the temptation to consume excessive amounts of food in one sitting.

3. Incorporating Nutrient-Dense Foods

Prioritize nutrient-dense diets, including fruits, vegetables, whole grains, and lean meats. These foods include critical vitamins, minerals, and antioxidants that promote liver function and contribute to general well-being.

4. Hydration

Cultivate the habit of remaining well-hydrated by taking a suitable amount of water throughout the day. Hydration is necessary for the optimum function of the liver, assisting in the detoxification process, and promoting general health.

5. Balanced Macronutrients

Strive for a balanced intake of carbs, proteins, and fats. A well-balanced diet ensures that your body obtains the key nutrients it needs for optimal functioning while supporting liver health.

6. Limiting Processed and Sugary Foods

Develop the practice of minimizing the intake of processed meals and added sugars. These can contribute to inflammation and hepatic fat storage. Opt for full, unprocessed meals to enhance liver health.

By implementing these healthy practices into your everyday life, you not only enhance liver health but also build a lifestyle that contributes to overall well-being.

These behaviors establish the basis for a robust and healthy liver, setting the stage for a life distinguished by vibrancy and enduring well-being.

The Journey Continues: Beyond the Cookbook

The transforming journey that began with the cookbook doesn't end with the last page. This chapter allows you to reflect on the progress you have made, praising the healthy habits you have adopted into your lifestyle. It extends the trip beyond the cookbook, enabling you to investigate new areas of well-being.

From regular physical exercise to stress management and comprehensive lifestyle choices, the chapter presents a path for maintaining the quest for maximum health.

As you embrace the "Fatty Liver Diet Cookbook" as a roadmap to well-being, remember that this is not simply a collection of recipes but a guide to a lifestyle that embraces balance, nourishment, and the delight of tasting tastes that support your liver and general health.

The road continues, and each dish is a step towards a future distinguished by energy, resilience, and a vibrant feeling of well-being.

CHAPTER 5

4-Week Meal Plan for a Healthy Fatty Liver Diet

This 28-day meal plan has been thoughtfully developed to not only excite your taste buds but also fuel your liver, supporting your quest for a healthier, more vibrant existence. Each day allows you to savor tasty, nutrient-dense meals while creating habits that contribute to the resilience of your liver.

Week 1

Day 1

Breakfast

- ✓ Scrambled eggs with spinach and tomatoes
- ✓ Whole-grain toast
- ✓ Green tea

Lunch

- ✓ Grilled chicken breast
- ✓ Quinoa salad with mixed veggies
- ✓ Apple slices

Dinner

- ✓ Baked salmon
- ✓ Steamed broccoli and carrots
- ✓ Brown rice

Snack

- ✓ Greek yogurt with a handful of berries

Day 2

Breakfast

- ✓ Oatmeal with sliced banana and a sprinkling of chia seeds
- ✓ Almond milk

Lunch

- ✓ Lentil soup
- ✓ Whole-grain roll
- ✓ Mixed green salad

Dinner

- ✓ Turkey stir-fry with colorful bell peppers
- ✓ Quinoa

Snack

- ✓ A handful of mixed nuts

Day 3

Breakfast

- ✓ Whole-grain pancakes with fresh berries
- ✓ Greek yogurt

Lunch

- ✓ Chickpea salad with cucumber, tomatoes, and feta
- ✓ Whole-grain pita

Dinner

- ✓ Grilled fish tacos with cabbage slaw
- ✓ Brown rice

Snack

- ✓ Sliced apple with almond butter

Day 4

Breakfast

- ✓ Smoothie with spinach, banana, berries, and almond milk

Lunch

- ✓ Chicken and vegetable stir-fry
- ✓ Quinoa

Dinner

- ✓ Baked cod with lemon and herbs
- ✓ Roasted sweet potatoes
- ✓ Steamed asparagus

Snack

- ✓ Carrot and cucumber sticks with hummus

Day 5

Breakfast

- ✓ Avocado toast with whole-grain bread
- ✓ Poached egg

Lunch

- ✓ Turkey and veggie wrap
- ✓ Mixed fruit salad

Dinner

- ✓ Quinoa-stuffed bell peppers
- ✓ Grilled zucchini

Snack

- ✓ Cottage cheese with pineapple chunks

Day 6

Breakfast

- ✓ Whole-grain waffles with strawberries and a splash of yogurt

Lunch

- ✓ Lentil and vegetable curry
- ✓ Brown rice

Dinner

- ✓ Grilled chicken breast with lemon and herbs
- ✓ Roasted Brussels sprouts
- ✓ Quinoa

Snack

- ✓ Mixed berries with a sprinkling of flaxseeds

Day 7

Breakfast

- ✓ Scrambled tofu with sautéed spinach and cherry tomatoes
- ✓ Whole-grain toast

Lunch

- ✓ Shrimp and broccoli stir-fry
- ✓ Quinoa

Dinner

- ✓ Baked tilapia with garlic and herbs
- ✓ Steamed green beans
- ✓ Sweet potato wedges

Snack

- ✓ A handful of walnuts

Week 2

Day 1

Breakfast

- ✓ Overnight oats with almond milk, chia seeds, and mixed fruit

Lunch

- ✓ Quinoa salad with black beans, corn, and avocado
- ✓ Whole-grain roll

Dinner

- ✓ Grilled veggie and chicken skewers
- ✓ Brown rice

Snack

- ✓ Sliced pear with a spread of almond butter

Day 2

Breakfast

- ✓ Whole-grain English muffin with smoked salmon and cream cheese

Lunch

- ✓ Chickpeas and vegetable stir-fry
- ✓ Quinoa

Dinner

- ✓ Baked chicken thighs with lemon and rosemary
- ✓ Roasted sweet potatoes
- ✓ Steamed broccoli

Snack

- ✓ Greek yogurt with a sprinkle of honey

Day 3

Breakfast

- ✓ Spinach and mushroom omelet
- ✓ Whole-grain toast

Lunch

- ✓ Tuna salad with mixed greens
- ✓ Whole-grain pita

Dinner

- ✓ Grilled prawns with garlic and herbs
- ✓ Quinoa
- ✓ Roasted Brussels sprouts

Snack

- ✓ Mixed fruit bowl

Day 4

Breakfast

- ✓ Whole-grain bread with smashed avocado and poached egg
- ✓ Fresh orange juice

Lunch

- ✓ Lentil and veggie wrap
- ✓ Mixed fruit salad

Dinner

- ✓ Baked cod with lemon and dill
- ✓ Quinoa
- ✓ Steamed asparagus

Snack

- ✓ Greek yogurt with a handful of almonds

Day 5

Breakfast

- ✓ Smoothie with kale, pineapple, banana, and coconut
  water

Lunch

- ✓ Turkey and vegetable stir-fry
- ✓ Brown rice

Dinner

- ✓ Grilled chicken breast with mango salsa
- ✓ Roasted sweet potatoes
- ✓ Steamed green beans

Snack

- ✓ Sliced apple with a sprinkling of cinnamon

Day 6

Breakfast

- ✓ Whole-grain pancakes with mixed berries and a dollop of yogurt

Lunch

- ✓ Chickpea and quinoa salad with cucumber and tomatoes
- ✓ Whole-grain pita

Dinner

- ✓ Baked fish with a honey mustard glaze
- ✓ Quinoa
- ✓ Grilled zucchini

Snack

- ✓ Cottage cheese with pineapple chunks

Day 7

Breakfast

- ✓ Avocado and tomato omelet
- ✓ Whole-grain bread

Lunch

- ✓ Shrimp and vegetable stir-fry
- ✓ Quinoa

Dinner

- ✓ Grilled veggie and tofu skewers
- ✓ Brown rice

Snack

- ✓ Mixed berries with a sprinkle of honey

Week 3

Day 1

Breakfast

- ✓ Whole-grain waffles with strawberries and a dollop of yogurt

Lunch

- ✓ Quinoa-stuffed bell peppers
- ✓ Mixed green salad

Dinner

- ✓ Baked tilapia with garlic and herbs
- ✓ Roasted Brussels sprouts
- ✓ Sweet potato wedges

Snack

A handful of walnuts

Day 2

Breakfast

- ✓ Overnight oats with almond milk, chia seeds, and mixed fruit

Lunch

- ✓ Quinoa salad with black beans, corn, and avocado
- ✓ Whole-grain roll

Dinner

- ✓ Grilled chicken thighs with lemon and rosemary
- ✓ Steamed broccoli
- ✓ Quinoa

Snack

- ✓ Sliced pear with a spread of almond butter

Day 3

Breakfast

- ✓ Whole-grain English muffin with smoked salmon and cream cheese

Lunch

- ✓ Tuna salad with mixed greens
- ✓ Whole-grain pita

Dinner

- ✓ Grilled shrimp with garlic and herbs
- ✓ Brown rice
- ✓ Roasted sweet potatoes

Snack

- ✓ Greek yogurt with a sprinkle of honey

Day 4

Breakfast

- ✓ Spinach and mushroom omelet
- ✓ Whole-grain bread

Lunch

- ✓ Chickpeas and vegetable stir-fry
- ✓ Quinoa

Dinner

- ✓ Baked chicken thighs with lemon and rosemary
- ✓ Steamed broccoli
- ✓ Quinoa

Snack

- ✓ Mixed fruit bowl

Day 5

Breakfast

- ✓ Whole-grain bread with smashed avocado and poached egg
- ✓ Fresh orange juice

Lunch

- ✓ Lentil and veggie wrap
- ✓ Mixed fruit salad

Dinner

- ✓ Baked cod with lemon and dill
- ✓ Quinoa
- ✓ Steamed asparagus

Snack

- ✓ Greek yogurt with a handful of almonds

Day 6

Breakfast

- ✓ Smoothie with kale, pineapple, banana, and coconut water

Lunch

- ✓ Turkey and vegetable stir-fry
- ✓ Brown rice

Dinner

- ✓ Grilled chicken breast with mango salsa
- ✓ Roasted sweet potatoes
- ✓ Steamed green beans

Snack

- ✓ Sliced apple with a sprinkling of cinnamon

Day 7

Breakfast

- ✓ Whole-grain pancakes with mixed berries and a dollop of yogurt

Lunch

- ✓ Chickpea and quinoa salad with cucumber and tomatoes
- ✓ Whole-grain pita

Dinner

- ✓ Baked fish with a honey mustard glaze
- ✓ Quinoa
- ✓ Grilled zucchini

Snack

- ✓ Cottage cheese with pineapple chunks

Week 4

Day | 1

Breakfast

- ✓ Avocado and tomato omelet
- ✓ Whole-grain bread

Lunch

- ✓ Shrimp and vegetable stir-fry
- ✓ Quinoa

Dinner

- ✓ Grilled veggie and tofu skewers
- ✓ Brown rice

Snack

- ✓ Mixed berries with a sprinkle of honey

Day 2

Breakfast

- ✓ Whole-grain waffles with strawberries and a dollop of yogurt

Lunch

- ✓ Quinoa-stuffed bell peppers
- ✓ Mixed green salad

Dinner

- ✓ Baked tilapia with garlic and herbs
- ✓ Roasted Brussels sprouts
- ✓ Sweet potato wedges

Snack

- ✓ A handful of walnuts

Day 3

Breakfast

- ✓ Overnight oats with almond milk, chia seeds, and mixed fruit

Lunch

- ✓ Quinoa salad with black beans, corn, and avocado
- ✓ Whole-grain roll

Dinner

- ✓ Grilled chicken thighs with lemon and rosemary
- ✓ Steamed broccoli
- ✓ Quinoa

Snack

- ✓ Sliced pear with a spread of almond butter

Day 4

Breakfast

- ✓ Whole-grain English muffin with smoked salmon and cream cheese

Lunch

- ✓ Tuna salad with mixed greens
- ✓ Whole-grain pita

Dinner

- ✓ Grilled shrimp with garlic and herbs
- ✓ Brown rice
- ✓ Roasted sweet potatoes

Snack

- ✓ Greek yogurt with a sprinkle of honey

Day 5

Breakfast

- ✓ Spinach and mushroom omelet
- ✓ Whole-grain bread

Lunch

- ✓ Chickpea and vegetable stir-fry
- ✓ Quinoa

Dinner

- ✓ Baked chicken thighs with lemon and rosemary
- ✓ Steamed broccoli
- ✓ Quinoa

Snack

- ✓ Mixed fruit bowl

Day 6

Breakfast

- ✓ Whole-grain bread with smashed avocado and poached egg
- ✓ Fresh orange juice

Lunch

- ✓ Lentil and veggie wrap
- ✓ Mixed fruit salad

Dinner

- ✓ Baked cod with lemon and dill
- ✓ Quinoa
- ✓ Steamed asparagus

Snack

- ✓ Greek yogurt with a handful of almonds

Day 7

Breakfast

- ✓ Smoothie with kale, pineapple, banana, and coconut water

Lunch

- ✓ Turkey and vegetable stir-fry
- ✓ Brown rice

Dinner

- ✓ Grilled chicken breast with mango salsa
- ✓ Roasted sweet potatoes
- ✓ Steamed green beans

Snack

- ✓ Sliced apple with a sprinkling of cinnamon

Congratulations on finishing this 4-week journey toward a better, liver-nourishing lifestyle. May the habits developed and the flavors experienced continue to add to your general well-being.

CHAPTER 6

Fatty Liver Diet Recipes

Unlock the potential of the "Fatty Liver Diet Cookbook" as you traverse its pages packed with delectable possibilities. This section leads you through the carefully picked recipes, each meant to excite your taste buds while nourishing your liver. From breakfast selections that launch your day to evening pleasures that bring joy to your tongue, the cookbook becomes your culinary compass on the route to well-being.

Breakfast Recipes

Start your day on a nutritious note with these delectable Fatty Liver Diet breakfast dishes. Packed with healthful ingredients that support liver health, these recipes are meant to launch your morning with a blast of taste and nutrition.

Avocado and Tomato Omelet

Ingredients

- ✓ 2 big eggs
- ✓ 1/2 avocado, sliced
- ✓ 1/2 cup cherry tomatoes, halved
- ✓ Salt and pepper to taste
- ✓ Fresh herbs for garnish (optional)

Preparation

1. Whisk eggs in a bowl and season with salt and pepper.
2. Pour the egg mixture into a prepared, non-stick skillet.
3. As the edges harden, add avocado slices and tomatoes.
4. Fold the omelet in half and cook until the eggs are fully set.
5. Garnish with fresh herbs, if desired.

Preparation Time: 10 minutes

Servings: 1

Berry and Chia Seed Parfait

Ingredients

- ✓ 1/2 cup Greek yogurt
- ✓ 1/4 cup mixed berries (blueberries, strawberries, raspberries)
- ✓ 2 tsp. chia seeds
- ✓ 1 tbsp. of honey or maple syrup (optional)
- ✓ Granola for topping (optional)

Preparation

1. In a glass, layer Greek yogurt, mixed berries, and chia seeds.
2. Repeat the layers until the glass is full.
3. Drizzle honey or maple syrup over top and sprinkle with granola if desired.

Preparation Time: 5 minutes (plus overnight for chia seeds to soak)

Servings: 1

Spinach and Mushroom Scramble

Ingredients

- ✓ 2 big eggs
- ✓ A handful of fresh spinach, chopped
- ✓ Half a cup of sliced
- ✓ 1 tbsp. of olive oil
- ✓ Salt and pepper to taste

Preparation

1. Heat olive oil in a pan and sauté mushrooms until soft.
2. Add chopped spinach and simmer until wilted.
3. Whisk eggs, season with salt and pepper, and pour into the skillet.
4. Scramble until the eggs are thoroughly cooked.

Preparation Time: 15 minutes

Servings: 1

Overnight Oats with Mixed Berries

Ingredients

1. Half a cup of rolled oats
2. Half a cup of almond milk
3. One-quarter cup of mixed berries (strawberries, blueberries, raspberries)
4. 1 tbsp. of chia seeds
5. 1 tbsp. of honey or maple syrup

Preparation

1. Combine oats, almond milk, mixed berries, and chia seeds in a container.
2. Stir thoroughly, cover, and chill overnight.
3. In the morning, sprinkle with honey or maple syrup before serving.

Preparation Time: 5 minutes (including overnight soaking)

Servings: 1

Whole-grain pancakes with Banana Slices

Ingredients

- ✓ Half a cup of whole-grain pancake mix
- ✓ Half a cup of almond milk
- ✓ Half banana, sliced
- ✓ 1 tbsp. nut butter (almond or peanut)
- ✓ 1 tsp. of honey (optional)

Preparation

1. Mix the pancake mix with almond milk until smooth.
2. Pour batter onto a hot griddle to create pancakes.
3. Top with banana slices, nut butter, and a sprinkle of honey if preferred.

Preparation Time: 15 minutes

Servings: 1-2

Scrambled Tofu Breakfast Burrito

Ingredients

- ✓ Half a cup of firm tofu crumbled
- ✓ One-quarter cup of black beans, washed and drained
- ✓ 2 tbsp. of salsa
- ✓ Whole-grain tortilla
- ✓ Fresh cilantro for garnish

Preparation

1. Sauté crumbled tofu in a pan until gently browned.
2. Add black beans and salsa, simmering until heated through.
3. Spoon the mixture onto a whole-grain tortilla, wrap, and top with cilantro.

Preparation Time: 10 minutes

Servings: 1

Greek Yogurt with Fruit Bowl

Ingredients

- ✓ Half a cup of Greek yogurt
- ✓ Half a cup of mixed fruit (kiwi, pineapple, mango)
- ✓ 1 tbsp. of chopped nuts (walnuts or almonds)
- ✓ 1 tsp. of honey

Preparation

- ✓ Spoon Greek yogurt into a bowl.
- ✓ Top with mixed fruit and chopped nuts.
- ✓ Drizzle with honey before serving.

Preparation Time: 5 minutes

Servings: 1

Whole-grain toast with Smashed Avocado and Poached Egg

Ingredients

- ✓ 1 piece whole-grain bread
- ✓ Half avocado, crushed
- ✓ 1 poached egg

✓ Salt and pepper to taste

Preparation

1. Toast the whole-grain bread to your taste.

2. Spread smashed avocado on the bread.

3. Top with a poached egg and season with salt and pepper.

Preparation Time: 10 minutes

Servings: 1

Quinoa Breakfast Bowl with Berries

Ingredients

✓ Half a cup of cooked quinoa

✓ One-quarter of a cup of Greek yogurt

✓ One-quarter cup of mixed berries (strawberries, blueberries, raspberries)

✓ 1 tbsp. of almond butter

Preparation

1. In a bowl, layer cooked quinoa, Greek yogurt, and mixed berries.
2. Drizzle with almond butter before serving.

Preparation Time: 10 minutes (if quinoa is pre-cooked)

Servings: 1

Smoothie with Spinach, Banana, and Almond Milk

Ingredients

- ✓ A handful of fresh spinach
- ✓ 1 banana
- ✓ Half a cup of almond milk
- ✓ 1 tbsp. of chia seeds
- ✓ Ice cubes (optional)

Preparation

1. Blend spinach, banana, almond milk, and chia seeds until smooth.
2. Add ice cubes if required and mix again.

Preparation Time: 5 minutes

Servings: 1

These Fatty Liver Diet breakfast recipes are not only delicious but also created to help your liver health. Incorporate these nutritious meals into your morning routine for a healthful start to the day.

Lunch Recipes

Lunch is a key part of your day, and these Fatty Liver Diet lunch meals are meant to give delicious alternatives that support liver health. Packed with nutrient-dense ingredients, these dishes offer a hearty midday meal that helps your overall well-being.

Grilled Chicken Salad with Lemon Vinaigrette

Ingredients

- ✓ 4 oz. grilled chicken breast, sliced
- ✓ Mixed greens (spinach, arugula, kale)

✓ Cherry tomatoes, halved

✓ Cucumber, sliced

✓ Red onion, thinly sliced

✓ Lemon vinaigrette dressing

Preparation

1. Grill the chicken until thoroughly done, then slice.

2. In a bowl, add mixed greens, cherry tomatoes, cucumber, and red onion.

3. Top with grilled chicken pieces and sprinkle with lemon vinaigrette.

Preparation Time: 15 minutes

Servings: 1

Lentil and Vegetable Wrap

Ingredients

✓ Half a cup of cooked lentils

✓ Whole-grain wrap

✓ Mixed veggies (bell peppers, cucumber, cherry tomatoes)

✓ Hummus for spreading

✓ Fresh parsley for garnish

Preparation

1. Spread hummus on the whole-grain wrap.

2. Layer cooked lentils and mixed veggies.

3. Garnish with fresh parsley and wrap it up.

Preparation Time: 10 minutes

Servings: 1

Quinoa Salad with Avocado and Chickpeas

Ingredients

✓ Half a cup of cooked quinoa

✓ 1/2 avocado, diced

✓ 1/4 cup chickpeas, washed and drained

✓ Cherry tomatoes, halved

✓ Cilantro for garnish

✓ Olive oil and lemon juice dressing

Preparation

1. In a bowl, add cooked quinoa, chopped avocado, chickpeas, and cherry tomatoes.
2. Drizzle with olive oil and a lemon juice dressing.
3. Garnish with cilantro before serving.

Preparation Time: 15 minutes

Servings: 1

Baked Salmon with Roasted Vegetables

Ingredients

- ✓ 4-ounce salmon fillet
- ✓ Mixed veggies (broccoli, carrots, bell peppers)
- ✓ Olive oil, garlic, and herbs for flavoring
- ✓ Lemon wedges for serving

Preparation

1. Season fish with olive oil, garlic, and herbs.
2. Place the fish on a baking sheet surrounded by mixed vegetables.

3. Bake until the salmon is cooked through and the veggies are roasted.

4. Serve with lemon wedges.

Preparation Time: 20 minutes

Servings: 1

Chickpea and Vegetable Stir-Fry

Ingredients

- ✓ Half a cup of cooked chickpeas
- ✓ Mixed veggies (bell peppers, broccoli, snap peas)
- ✓ Soy sauce with ginger for stir-frying
- ✓ Brown rice for serving

Preparation

1. Stir-fry mixed veggies in a skillet with soy sauce and ginger.

2. Add cooked chickpeas and continue to stir-fry until heated through.

3. Serve over a bed of brown rice.

Preparation Time: 15 minutes

Servings: 1

Turkey and Quinoa Stuffed Bell Peppers

Ingredients

- ✓ Half a cup of cooked quinoa
- ✓ Lean ground turkey
- ✓ Bell peppers, halved
- ✓ Tomato sauce for topping
- ✓ Italian herbs for spice

Preparation

1. Cook ground turkey and combine it with cooked quinoa and Italian herbs.
2. Stuff bell peppers with the turkey and quinoa mixture.
3. Top with tomato sauce and bake until the peppers are soft.

Preparation Time: 30 minutes

Servings: 2

Grilled Shrimp Salad with Citrus Dressing

Ingredients

- ✓ 4 ounces grilled shrimp
- ✓ Mixed greens (arugula, spinach, and watercress)
- ✓ Grapefruit segments
- ✓ Avocado, sliced
- ✓ Citrus dressing

Preparation

1. Grill shrimp until done and leave aside.
2. In a bowl, add mixed greens, grapefruit pieces, and avocado.
3. Top with grilled shrimp and sprinkle with citrus dressing.

Preparation Time: 20 minutes

Servings: 1

Lentil and Vegetable Curry

Ingredients

- ✓ 1/2 cup cooked lentils
- ✓ Mixed veggies (zucchini, carrots, peas)
- ✓ Curry sauce (coconut milk, curry paste)
- ✓ Brown rice for serving

Preparation

1. Cook mixed veggies in a pan till soft.
2. Add cooked lentils and curry sauce, boiling until heated through.
3. Serve over brown rice.

Preparation Time: 25 minutes

Servings: 1

Tuna Salad Lettuce Wraps

Ingredients

- ✓ Canned tuna, drained
- ✓ Greek yogurt for binding
- ✓ Celery, finely chopped
- ✓ Lettuce leaves for wrapping
- ✓ Cherry tomatoes for garnish

Preparation

1. Mix tuna with Greek yogurt and diced celery.
2. Spoon the tuna mixture onto lettuce leaves.
3. Garnish with cherry tomatoes and wrap.

Preparation Time: 10 minutes

Servings: 1

Mediterranean Quinoa Bowl

Ingredients

- ✓ 1/2 cup cooked quinoa
- ✓ Hummus for spreading
- ✓ Cherry tomatoes, halved
- ✓ Cucumber, diced
- ✓ Kalamata olives, sliced
- ✓ Feta cheese for topping

Preparation

1. Spread hummus on the base of a bowl.
2. Layer with cooked quinoa, cherry tomatoes, cucumber, and Kalamata olives.
3. Top with crumbled feta cheese.

Preparation Time: 15 minutes

Servings: 1

These Fatty Liver Diet lunch meals offer a range of tastes and textures while favoring nutrients that help liver function. Enjoy these nutritious dishes as part of your lunchtime routine for a delicious and fulfilling lunch.

Dinner Recipes

End your day on a healthy and appetizing note with these Fatty Liver Diet supper dishes. Designed to support liver health, these recipes offer healthful ingredients and delectable combinations that make for a full and fulfilling evening meal.

Baked Cod with Lemon and Dill

Ingredients

- ✓ 6-ounce cod fillet
- ✓ Fresh lemon juice
- ✓ Fresh dill, chopped
- ✓ Olive oil
- ✓ Garlic powder
- ✓ Salt and pepper

Preparation

1. Preheat the oven and arrange the fish on a baking sheet.
2. Drizzle with olive oil and lemon juice.
3. Season with garlic powder, salt, and pepper.

4. Bake until the fish is cooked through.

5. Sprinkle with chopped dill before serving.

Preparation Time: 20 minutes

Servings: 1

Grilled Chicken Breast with Mango Salsa

Ingredients

- ✓ 1 boneless, skinless chicken breast
- ✓ Ripe mango, diced
- ✓ Red onion, finely chopped
- ✓ Fresh cilantro, chopped
- ✓ Lime juice
- ✓ Salt and pepper

Preparation

1. Grill the chicken breast until thoroughly done.

2. In a bowl, add chopped mango, red onion, cilantro, and lime juice.

3. Top the cooked chicken with mango salsa.

Preparation Time: 25 minutes

Servings: 1

Quinoa-Stuffed Bell Peppers

Ingredients

- ✓ Bell peppers, halved
- ✓ 1/2 cup cooked quinoa
- ✓ Black beans, washed and drained
- ✓ Corn kernels
- ✓ Cumin and chili powder
- ✓ Tomato sauce

Preparation

1. Preheat the oven and place bell peppers in a baking dish.
2. Mix cooked quinoa, black beans, corn, cumin, and chili powder.
3. Stuff bell peppers with the quinoa mixture.
4. Pour tomato sauce over the top and bake until the peppers are soft.

Preparation Time: 30 minutes

Servings: 2

Turkey and Vegetable Stir-Fry

Ingredients

- ✓ Lean ground turkey
- ✓ Mixed veggies (broccoli, bell peppers, snap peas)
- ✓ Soy sauce with ginger
- ✓ Brown rice

Preparation

1. Cook ground turkey in a pan until browned.
2. Add mixed veggies, soy sauce, and ginger.
3. Stir-fry until veggies are soft.
4. Serve over a bed of brown rice.

Preparation Time: 20 minutes

Servings: 1

Grilled Vegetable and Tofu Skewers

Ingredients

- ✓ Firm tofu, cubed
- ✓ Mixed veggies (zucchini, cherry tomatoes, mushrooms)
- ✓ Olive oil with balsamic vinegar
- ✓ Italian herbs
- ✓ Skewers

Preparation

1. Thread tofu and mixed veggies onto skewers.
2. Mix olive oil, balsamic vinegar, and Italian herbs.
3. Brush skewers with the mixture and cook until veggies are tender.

Preparation Time: 25 minutes

Servings: 2

Chickpea and Vegetable Curry

Ingredients

- ✓ Half a cup of cooked chickpeas
- ✓ Mixed veggies (zucchini, carrots, peas)
- ✓ Curry sauce (coconut milk, curry paste)
- ✓ Brown rice

Preparation

1. Cook mixed veggies in a pan till soft.
2. Add cooked chickpeas and curry sauce, boiling until heated through.
3. Serve over brown rice.

Preparation Time: 25 minutes

Servings: 1

Spinach and Mushroom Stuffed Chicken Breast

Ingredients:

- ✓ Boneless, skinless chicken breast
- ✓ Fresh spinach
- ✓ Mushrooms, sliced
- ✓ Garlic and onion, minced
- ✓ Olive oil
- ✓ Italian herbs

Preparation

1. Preheat the oven and butterfly the chicken breast.
2. Sauté spinach, mushrooms, garlic, and onion in olive oil.
3. Stuff the chicken breast with the sautéed mixture.
4. Bake until the chicken is cooked through.

Preparation Time: 30 minutes

Servings: 1

Baked Salmon with Herb Crust

Ingredients

- ✓ 6 oz. of salmon fillet
- ✓ Dijon mustard
- ✓ Fresh herbs (parsley, dill, chives)
- ✓ Lemon zest
- ✓ Olive oil
- ✓ Salt and pepper

Preparation

1. Preheat the oven and arrange the fish on a baking sheet.
2. Mix Dijon mustard, chopped herbs, lemon zest, and olive oil.
3. Spread the herb mixture over the fish.
4. Bake until the fish is cooked through.

Preparation Time: 20 minutes

Servings: 1

Quinoa Salad with Black Beans and Avocado

Ingredients

- ✓ 1/2 cup cooked quinoa
- ✓ Black beans, washed and drained
- ✓ Avocado, diced
- ✓ Cherry tomatoes, halved
- ✓ Lime juice
- ✓ Cilantro for garnish

Preparation

1. In a bowl, add cooked quinoa, black beans, chopped avocado, and cherry tomatoes.
2. Drizzle with lime juice and garnish with cilantro.

Preparation Time: 15 minutes

Servings: 1

Shrimp and Broccoli Stir-Fry

Ingredients

- ✓ Shrimp, peeled and deveined
- ✓ Broccoli florets
- ✓ Soy sauce with ginger
- ✓ Brown rice

Preparation

1. Stir-fry shrimp and broccoli in a pan with soy sauce and ginger.
2. Cook until shrimp are pink and broccoli is soft.
3. Serve over a bed of brown rice.

Preparation Time: 20 minutes

Servings: 1

These Fatty Liver Diet supper dishes offer a broad selection of flavors and textures, ensuring that your evening meals are both delicious and supportive of liver health. Enjoy these healthful recipes as you wind down your day with tasty, wholesome selections.

Snack Recipes

Snacking doesn't have to be synonymous with guilt, especially when you're on a Fatty Liver Diet. These snack recipes are not only delicious but also designed to support liver health. From crunchy bites to savory treats, each recipe is crafted with wholesome ingredients to keep you satisfied and nourished between meals.

Roasted Chickpeas with Turmeric

Ingredients

- ✓ One can (15 oz.) of chickpeas, drained and rinsed
- ✓ One tbsp. of olive oil
- ✓ One tsp. of turmeric
- ✓ Half tsp. of cumin
- ✓ Salt and pepper to taste

Preparation

1. Preheat the oven to 400°F (200°C).
2. Pat chickpeas dry and toss with olive oil, turmeric, cumin, salt, and pepper.

✓ Spread on a baking sheet and roast for 25-30 minutes until crispy.

Preparation Time: 30 minutes

Servings: 4

Greek Yogurt Parfait with Berries

Ingredients

✓ One cup of Greek yogurt

✓ Half cup mixed berries (blueberries, strawberries)

✓ Two tbsp. of granola

✓ Drizzle of honey (optional)

Preparation

1. In a glass, layer Greek yogurt, mixed berries, and granola.

2. Repeat the layers until the glass is filled.

3. Drizzle with honey if desired.

Preparation Time: 5 minutes

Servings: 1

Avocado and Tomato Salsa

Ingredients

- ✓ One ripe avocado, diced
- ✓ One cup of cherry tomatoes, diced
- ✓ One-quarter cup of red onion, finely chopped
- ✓ Fresh cilantro, chopped
- ✓ Lime juice
- ✓ Salt and pepper to taste

Preparation

1. In a bowl, combine diced avocado, tomatoes, red onion, and cilantro.
2. Drizzle with lime juice and season with salt and pepper.
3. Serve with whole-grain crackers or veggie sticks.

Preparation Time: 10 minutes

Servings: 2

Nut and Seed Trail Mix

Ingredients

- ✓ Half a cup of almonds
- ✓ Half a cup of walnuts
- ✓ One-quarter cup of pumpkin seeds
- ✓ One-quarter cup of dried cranberries
- ✓ One-quarter tsp. of cinnamon
- ✓ Pinch of sea salt

Preparation

1. Mix almonds, walnuts, pumpkin seeds, dried cranberries, cinnamon, and sea salt in a bowl.
2. Portion into snack-sized servings.

Preparation Time: 5 minutes

Servings: 4

Hummus and Veggie Sticks

Ingredients

- ✓ One cup of hummus
- ✓ Carrot sticks, cucumber slices, and bell pepper strips for dipping

Preparation

1. Arrange hummus in a bowl.
2. Prepare carrot sticks, cucumber slices, and bell pepper strips for dipping.

Preparation Time: 5 minutes

Servings: 2

Cottage Cheese with Pineapple

Ingredients

- ✓ One cup of low-fat cottage cheese
- ✓ Half a cup of fresh pineapple chunks
- ✓ Mint leaves for garnish (optional)

Preparation

1. Spoon cottage cheese into a bowl.

2. Top with fresh pineapple chunks.

3. Garnish with mint leaves if desired.

Preparation Time: 5 minutes

Servings: 1

Zucchini Chips with Sea Salt

Ingredients

- ✓ Two zucchinis, thinly sliced
- ✓ One tbsp. of olive oil
- ✓ Sea salt to taste

Preparation

1. Preheat the oven to 225°F (110°C).

2. Toss zucchini slices with olive oil and arrange on a baking sheet.

3. Sprinkle with sea salt and bake for 2 hours until crisp.

Preparation Time: 2 hours

Servings: 2

Apple Slices with Almond Butter

Ingredients

- ✓ One apple, sliced
- ✓ Two tbsp. of almond butter

Preparation

1. Arrange apple slices on a plate.
2. Serve with almond butter for dipping.

Preparation Time: 5 minutes

Servings: 1

Quinoa and Black Bean Salad Cups

Ingredients

- ✓ Half a cup of cooked quinoa
- ✓ One-quarter cup of black beans, rinsed and drained
- ✓ Cherry tomatoes, halved
- ✓ Fresh parsley, chopped

✓ Lemon vinaigrette dressing

Preparation

1. In a bowl, mix quinoa, black beans, cherry tomatoes, and parsley.
2. Drizzle with lemon vinaigrette dressing.
3. Spoon into small cups for a portable snack.

Preparation Time: 15 minutes

Servings: 2

Baked Sweet Potato Fries

Ingredients

✓ Two sweet potatoes, cut into fries

✓ One tbsp. of olive oil

✓ Half tsp. of paprika

✓ One-quarter tsp. of garlic powder

✓ Salt and pepper to taste

Preparation

1. Preheat the oven to 425°F (220°C).
2. Toss sweet potato fries with olive oil, paprika, garlic powder, salt, and pepper.
3. Spread on a baking sheet and bake for 25-30 minutes until crispy.

Preparation Time: 30 minutes

Servings: 4

These Fatty Liver Diet snack recipes offer a variety of flavors and textures, ensuring your snack time is not only enjoyable but also supportive of your liver health. Incorporate these delicious options into your routine for a satisfying and nourishing snacking experience.

Smoothie Recipes

Kick start your day or enjoy a refreshing snack with these Fatty Liver Diet smoothie recipes. Packed with wholesome ingredients, these delicious blends are tailored to support liver health while tantalizing your taste buds.

From vibrant greens to antioxidant-rich fruits, each smoothie is a nourishing delight that contributes to your overall well-being.

Green Goddess Detox Smoothie

Ingredients

- ✓ One cup of spinach
- ✓ Half of cucumber, peeled and sliced
- ✓ Half of green apple, cored
- ✓ Half lemon, juiced
- ✓ One cup of coconut water
- ✓ Ice cubes

Preparation

1. Combine spinach, cucumber, green apple, lemon juice, and coconut water in a blender.
2. Blend until smooth.
3. Add ice cubes and blend again.

Preparation Time: 5 minutes

Servings: 1

Berry Bliss Liver Cleanse Smoothie

Ingredients

- ✓ Half a cup of blueberries
- ✓ Half a cup of raspberries
- ✓ Half cup of strawberries, hulled
- ✓ One tbsp. of chia seeds
- ✓ One cup of almond milk
- ✓ Ice cubes

Preparation

1. Blend blueberries, raspberries, strawberries, chia seeds, and almond milk until smooth.
2. Add ice cubes and blend again.

Preparation Time: 5 minutes

Servings: 1

Tropical Turmeric Twist Smoothie

Ingredients

- ✓ Half a cup of pineapple chunks
- ✓ Half mango, peeled and diced
- ✓ One tsp. of turmeric powder
- ✓ One tbsp. of flaxseeds
- ✓ One cup of coconut water
- ✓ Ice cubes

Preparation

1. Blend pineapple, mango, turmeric powder, flaxseeds, and coconut water until smooth.
2. Add ice cubes and blend again.

Preparation Time: 5 minutes

Servings: 1

Citrus Surge Liver Boost Smoothie

Ingredients

- ✓ One orange, peeled and segmented
- ✓ Half grapefruit, peeled and segmented
- ✓ Half lemon, juiced
- ✓ One tbsp. of hemp seeds
- ✓ One cup of water
- ✓ Ice cubes

Preparation

1. Blend orange, grapefruit, lemon juice, hemp seeds, and water until smooth.
2. Add ice cubes and blend again.

Preparation Time: 5 minutes

Servings: 1

Kale & Kiwi Revitalizing Smoothie

Ingredients

- ✓ One cup of kale stems removed
- ✓ Two kiwis, peeled and sliced
- ✓ Half banana
- ✓ One tbsp. of pumpkin seeds
- ✓ One cup of coconut water
- ✓ Ice cubes

Preparation

1. Blend kale, kiwis, banana, pumpkin seeds, and coconut water until smooth.
2. Add ice cubes and blend again.

Preparation Time: 5 minutes

Servings: 1

Minty Melon Liver Refresh Smoothie

Ingredients

- ✓ One cup of honeydew melon, diced
- ✓ Half cucumber, peeled and sliced
- ✓ A handful of fresh mint leaves
- ✓ One tbsp. of chia seeds
- ✓ One cup of water
- ✓ Ice cubes

Preparation

1. Blend honeydew melon, cucumber, mint leaves, chia seeds, and water until smooth.
2. Add ice cubes and blend again.

Preparation Time: 5 minutes

Servings: 1

Blue Zone Berry Blast Smoothie

Ingredients

- ✓ Half a cup of acai berries (frozen)
- ✓ Half a cup of pomegranate seeds
- ✓ Half a cup of blackberries
- ✓ One tbsp. of flaxseeds
- ✓ One cup of almond milk
- ✓ Ice cubes

Preparation

1. Blend acai berries, pomegranate seeds, blackberries, flaxseeds, and almond milk until smooth.
2. Add ice cubes and blend again.

Preparation Time: 5 minutes

Servings: 1

Pineapple Turmeric Elixir Smoothie

Ingredients

- ✓ One cup of pineapple chunks
- ✓ Half tsp. of turmeric powder
- ✓ Half tsp. of ginger, grated
- ✓ One tbsp. of chia seeds
- ✓ One cup of coconut water
- ✓ Ice cubes

Preparation

1. Blend pineapple, turmeric powder, ginger, chia seeds, and coconut water until smooth.
2. Add ice cubes and blend again.

Preparation Time: 5 minutes

Servings: 1

Golden Beet Energizer Smoothie

Ingredients

- ✓ One golden beet, peeled and diced
- ✓ Half cup of strawberries, hulled
- ✓ Half a cup of raspberries
- ✓ One tbsp. of hemp seeds
- ✓ One cup of water
- ✓ Ice cubes

Preparation

1. Blend golden beet, strawberries, raspberries, hemp seeds, and water until smooth.
2. Add ice cubes and blend again.

Preparation Time: 5 minutes

Servings: 1

Chocolate Avocado Bliss Smoothie

Ingredients

- ✓ Half avocado, peeled and diced
- ✓ One tbsp. of cacao powder
- ✓ One tbsp. of almond butter
- ✓ One tbsp. of chia seeds
- ✓ One cup of almond milk
- ✓ Ice cubes

Preparation

1. Blend avocado, cacao powder, almond butter, chia seeds, and almond milk until smooth.
2. Add ice cubes and blend again.

Preparation Time: 5 minutes

Servings: 1

These Fatty Liver Diet smoothie recipes are not only a treat for your taste buds but also a nourishing way to support your liver health. Incorporate these vibrant blends into your routine for a delightful and nutritious boost anytime during the day.

CONCLUSION

As we close the pages of the "Fatty Liver Diet Cookbook," it's not just a culinary trip we've gone on but a profound investigation of the symbiotic link between food and liver function. In our quest to make tasty and wholesome meals, we've unearthed the transformative potential that mindful eating can have on our well-being.

Fatty liver disease is a frequent disorder that demands more than just medical intervention; it calls for a holistic approach that begins in the kitchen.

This cookbook has been more than a collection of recipes—it's a guide, a companion, and a source of empowerment for individuals trying to take care of their liver health.

We started by grasping the significance of fatty liver disease, recognizing its influence on our bodies, and realizing the essential role that nutrition plays in both its management and prevention.

The meals offered here are not simply gourmet delights; they are nutritional tools meant to nourish and heal. From the basic guidance to a healthy liver lifestyle to the deep examination of culinary remedies for fatty liver wellbeing, each chapter has been a step towards developing a healthier, more mindful connection with our bodies.

The 4-week meal plan offered in the later half of this book serves as a practical roadmap—a real, day-by-day guide to adopting the ideas addressed. It's more than a meal plan; it's a commitment to one's health, a vow to prioritize nourishment, and an awareness that every mouthful is a chance to cultivate well-being.

As you begin this gastronomic adventure, remember that the route towards a healthy liver is not a sprint but a marathon. Every dish, every ingredient, and every conscious moment in the kitchen adds to your overall health.

Beyond the cookbook, let this be a starting point for a lifestyle that celebrates balance, welcomes nourishment, and acknowledges the fundamental relationship between what we eat and how we live.

May this cookbook serve as a daily reminder that taking care of your liver is an act of self-love, and with every healthy meal, you're investing in a future of energy and well-being. Here's to your health, your adventure, and the many wonderful chapters that lie ahead.

Cheers to a happy and healthy life!